PREFACE

Ayurveda is a system of medicine with historical roots in the Indian subcontinent. Globalized and modernized practices derived from Ayurveda traditions are a type of complementary or alternative medicine .In countries beyond India, Ayurveda therapies and practices have been integrated in general wellness applications and in some cases in medical use.

Some scholars assert that Ayurveda originated in prehistoric times and that some of the concepts of Ayurveda have existed from the time of the Indus Valley Civilization or even earlier. Ayurveda developed significantly during the Vedic period and later some of the non-Vedic systems such as Buddhism and Jainism also developed medical concepts and practices that appear in the classical Ayurveda texts. Doṣha balance is emphasized, and suppressing natural urges is considered unhealthy and claimed to lead to illness. Ayurveda treatises describe three elemental doṣhas viz. vata, pitta(acidity) and kapha, and state that equality of the doṣhas results in health, while inequality results in disease.

Prevention is always better than cure. Through this book you will understand the basic reasons of various diseases. With this knowledge you can maintain your health and can prevent various diseases.

In this book we are also giving various Ayurveda's home remedies for recovery of disease and to tips to maintain proper balance of Vata, Pitta (acidity) and kapha. Before applying home remedy, consult your doctor.

Wish you a healthy and long life. Wish you a happy reading.

Warm Regards

(BE Production)

From Latur, Maharashtra ,India

shivshankar.sangale@gmail.com

Table of Contents

THE SCIENCE OF AYURVEDA AND THE THREE DOSHAS VATA,PITTA,KAPHA

The ancient science of Ayurveda is the oldest known form of health care in the world. Often called the mother of all healing, it originated in India some 5000 or more years ago.

Ayurveda is widely practiced all over the world and
is recognized by WHO (world health organization)

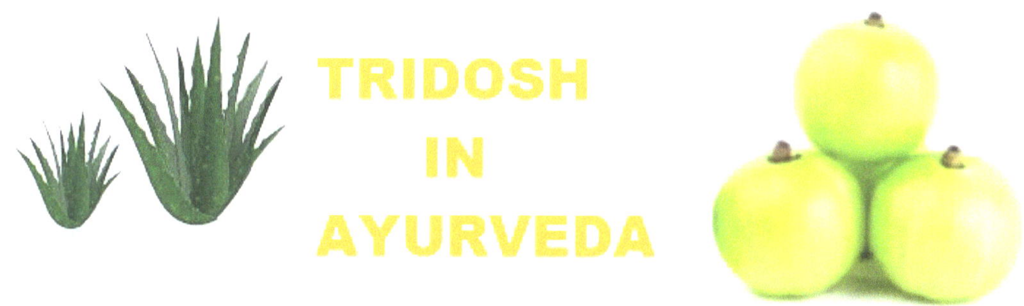

Ayur means long life & veda means knowledge or science. In Ayurveda diagnosis is done by observation, touch and questioning.

Cures chronic and stubborn diseases by its deep rooted treatment procedures and drugs. Ayurvedic medicines are derived from herbs, plants,
flowers, fruits etc. It is harmless, non-toxic and self-contained.

Ayurveda is a medical system that deals not only with body but with the mind and spirit as well.The fundamental aim of ayurvedic therapy is to restore the balance between the 3 humours or dosha (**VATA, PITTA, KAPHA**) and coordination of body, mind, and consciousness.

Health is not just absence of disease,balance of Vat, Pitta & cough is Health
Imbalance of these three is Disease.

Our body is made of five elements, which are as below.

Air: Gaseous form of matter which is in motion

Fire: Power to transform solids – liquids – gas and back again
Water: Characterizes change and represents the liquid state – unstable
Earth: Represents the solid state of matter – stable
Ether: Space in which everything happens

What are Doshas?

Doshas are defined as energetic principles that govern physiological and psychological functions of the body.

There are three Doshas:**Vata, Pitta** and **Kapha**
Health exists when there is a balance between these three. Unbalance of these three is called as disease.

Theory of Tri Doshas

Vata

Related to Air and Ether.
Principle of movement, physical and mental function
Directs nerve impulses, circulation,respiration, elimination and degeneration

Pitta (acidity)

Related to Fire and Water
Principle of digestion, absorption assimilation and transformation
Transforms food into nutrients,Related to Metabolism in the digestive system.

Kapha

Related to Water and Earth
Principle of structure &solidity bonding, cohesiveness, growth and lubrication,
Growth and protection,Mucosal lining of the stomach, Protection of the brain and back bone.

According to predominance of basic elements, persons are also divided in three types

VAT	PITTA (ACIDITY)	KAPHA
EARTH + WATER	FIRE + WATER	AIR + SPACE
Person is thin built	Medium built	Broad and stout built
Cold hands and feet	Warm hands and feet	Adaptable, dislikes wet and cold temp; cool hands
Dry skin	Oily skin	Thick, moist, pale and cool skin
Frizzy hair	Fine hair	Thick, oily and lustrous hair
Weak colonic digestion	Acne, cold sores, fungal infection	Digestive disorders, mucous formation
Extreme sensitivity to weather; tendency to be nervous and worry; enthusiastic	Like cooler temperatures; tendency to be angry and irritable; strong intellect	Nature is calm and stable; excellent memory, tendency towards inactivity; greed and attachment
Food to Counteract Doshas		
Amla, Non refined Sunflower oil	Amla, Pea Nuts, Jaggery,Bottle Guard, Tulsi leaves, Alo vera juice, Human saliva,sprouts	Amla, Ghee,Clove,Ginger

	Major Diseases	
Joint pen, knee pain Ankle pain etc.	All diseases which occur in stomach, lever, heart ,kidney ,small & large intestine etc. Diabetes	Disease of respiratory system, brain, ENT Problems ,BONES etc.

Every person contains all three doshas.
However, the proportion varies according to the individual and usually one or two doshas predominate. Within each person the doshas are continually interacting with one another and with the doshas in all the nature.
This explains why people can have much in common but also have an endless variety of individual differences in the way they behave and respond to their Environment.

These three dohsa have their specific timings in a day. In that time that particular dosha dominates other two.

6 am to 11 am – Kapha
11 am to 5 pm- Pitta
5 pm to 9pm – Vat

Night
9 to 12 Midnight-Kapha
12 to 3 am- Pitta
3 to 6 am – Vata

Seasonal effects on Dosha

	Vata	Pitta	Kapha
Late Winters			Accumulation
Spring			Aggravation
Summer	Accumulation		Mitigation
Rains	Aggravation	Accumulation	
Autumn	Mitigation	Aggravation	
Early winter		Mitigation	

TOP SECRET OF DRINKING WATER

Best drinking water

Rain water which is collected before dropping on earth is best as compared to other water. It does not have any expiry date. Second best is river water which is connected to glacier. Next is pond water which stores rain water. Next is bore well water & last is water supplied by Municipal Corporation.

Try to collect & store rain water under underground tanks, or send it to bore well. Lime stone is very helpful for purifying such water.

It is always better to use boiled water for drinking, it will be better than water purifier & RO water. Purifier and RO, removes necessary minerals from water.

Water Drinking Timings As Per Ayurveda

Water should be always sipped. Animal and birds like lion, sparrow sip the water. Do not drink water in standing position. In morning after wake up, water should be sipped before cleaning your mouth. It captures saliva, which is alkaline in nature and is very useful for our body. It reduces acidity & tries to make our stomach neutral.

Water should be taken before 1 to 1.5 hours of meal. After meal you can take water after 1 to 1.5 hr. In cold regions like Himalaya,USA, CANANADA,UK etc.water should be taken after 2 to 2.5 hours.

If you immediately drink water after meal, it will slow down digestion. It can result in decay of food, producing harmful gases.

Which can lead to lot of diseases like Acidity, Constipation, Alsar, Mulvadh, cancer etc.

Between meals at junction of two different foods, you can take 2 spoon of water (20 ml). Junction means you have finished first food (made of wheat) & now going to eat second food (rice) at that moment, 2 spoons of water can be taken to clear throat.

Quantity of drinking water

In a day maximum a person should drink water up to 10% of his weight. Minimum should be 10 times of his food weight. Suppose a person eat 500 gram of food in a day. He should drink minimum 5 liters of water in a day.

Never drink cold water

Cold water is very dangerous to health. Never drink ice mixed water or water of refrigerator. It can cool down your stomach, which will also cool down your heart & brain.

Body will try to maintain its temperature, in order to heat your stomach; it will absorb temperature from blood. More blood will flow to stomach; it can reduce blood supply to brain and heart.

If it happens always, it can lead to diseases like brain hemorrhage, paralysis, heart attack, constipation etc.

Do not eat ice cream after warm meal. It should be at normal body temperature.

Liquids that can be taken immediately after meal.

After breakfast, fruit juice can be taken. After lunch butter milk can be taken. After sunset milk is recommended.

TOP SECRETS OF FOOD

You are what you eat

Food has vibrations & the person who cooked your food, his thoughts also affects food vibrations. Try same food (1) At your house made by mother (2) At restaurant (3) At some mandir,Gurudawara (4) Same food cooked by servant.

All will give you different vibrations; it will give different impact on your thoughts. Because consciousness of person who is cooking is different. Mother who is cooking, he has full of love & affection for her child and family. At restaurant they are cooking for profit & selling. At Mandir, Gurudwara, food is cooked to do function of good; it is Prasad of god for their children's. So right consciousness will give write energy to our mind and body. So house wives and mothers should cook food only when they are fresh and energetic and have good energy.

Always prefer food of your own house cooked by your family than restaurant. Suppose you are visiting at some place, environment is very good & clean, but there is chance that you feel, some negative vibrations, test of food is secondary. While eating our mind should be also very calm, you should not eat while watching TV, reading or doing some another work.

Human thoughts also affect growth of plants. Scientific experiment is done on this subject, same plant, same seeds, and same soil; only the person who is giving water to plant is changed. Plant which was watered by criminal has less growth. Plant watered by normal human has some extra growth, and plants which are watered by noble person who have attachment with plant, got highest growth.

The plant is living thing and its energy can be measured. Energy is in the form of aura. It can be observed with callier photography. The observations of photography are as below.

    (1) Fruits have highest energy
    (2) Sprouts have second highest energy level.
    (3) Vegetables have third energy level.
    (4) Cooked food like dal, roti, rice has fourth energy level.

In Japan some scientist has done experiment on water by giving different thoughts on them. They found that with positive thoughts, the molecular structure becomes very beautiful & with negative thoughts they found that molecular structure of water gets disturbed.

In human body water is the main content. So be positive about all humans who are in touch with you, they should feel positive vibrations, when they come in your contact. Then only you will get positive work & results from them.

Do you fill petrol in diesel vehicle??

__HUMAN BODY IS MADE FOR VEG FOOD & NOT FOR NON VEG FOOD!! NOT UNDERSTOOD!! READ THE FOLLOWING PARAGRAPH.__

Please note the difference of nails, canine teeth's in vegetarian & non vegetarian animals, you will understand human comes under vegetarian category

Also note water drinking style of non-vegetarians & vegetarian animals. Lion, tiger, dogs etc. drink water by their tongue. And cow, horse, goat all these animals drink water by their mouth. Human also use their mouth, to drink water, it indicates that man is vegetarian animal.

Saliva of vegetarian animals is alkaline; in non-vegetarian animals it is highly acidic. Human saliva is alkaline; it clearly indicates that humans are vegetarian.

In non-vegetarian animals, their stomach contains very high quantity of acid, in order to digest animal food. In vegetarian animals their stomach contains very less acid. It also indicates than human comes under vegetarian category.

In vegetarian animals small intestine is around 20 to 22 feet's long but in non-vegetarian animals it is around 5 to 6 feet's long only. It also indicates that human body is made for veg food only.

Bile secretion is very less in vegetarian animals, in non-vegetarian animals bile secretion is very high as they consume more fat, it also indicates that all humans are vegetarians.

Vegetarian animals secret sweat to cool down, non-vegetarian animals suck more air from their mouth to cool down their body temperature. It also indicates that all humans come under vegetarian category.

VEGETARIAN FOOD	NON- VEGETARIAN FOOD
Vegetarian peoples live longer.	Non vegetarian peoples live shorter.
Vegetarian diet is healthier than non-vegetarian. Vegetarian diet prevent heart disease or help in reversing in heart diseases, it also reduces risk of cancer. Low fat vegetarian diet is most effective to stop progression, of coronary artery disease, or prevent it entirely.	Animal products are reach source of saturated fat, which increase chance of coronary heart disease. Cardiovascular disease kills around 7 Lakhs Americans, per annum and is leading cause of death in USA.
Low fact and low cholesterol food like leafy vegetables, apples, help to reduce extra body weight. And help to maintain your correct body weight. The fact that plant source do not have cholesterol is enough to become vegetarian.	Peoples who are non-vegetarian they are more prone to obesity.
Veg food has low sodium & low fat, so less chances of hypertension than non-vegetarian.	Non- vegetarian have high chances of hypertension.

Vegetarian diet is healthful, because vegetarians do not eat animal fat & cholesterol, and eat more fiber and antioxidant reach food. Veg food keeps immune system strong and keeps away mental disorder.	It reduces immunity, attracts more diseases.

VEGETARIAN FOOD	NON- VEGETARIAN FOOD
Veg food is more approachable to insulin.	Non vegetarian have twice chance of getting diabetes disease.
Less chances of getting kidney stone & gall stone	Non veg diet is reach in protein, sometimes excess amount of protein can lead body to exert more amounts of calcium, oxalate, uric acid, and it can lead to kidney stone and gall stone.

Vegetarian gets natural protection against prostate, stomach, lungs & breast cancer, colon cancer.	Non vegetarian has more risk of colon cancer.

Research by "spiritual sicinece research foundation"

According to spiritual science, entire universe is made of 3 basic subtle components which are (1) Sattva (2) Raja (3) Tama,

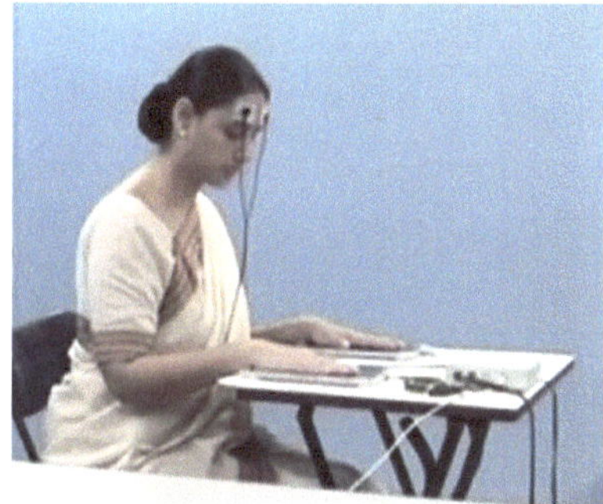

Sattva represent spiritual purity and knowledge. Raja represents action and passion. Tama represents ignorance and inertia.

Electrosomatographic scanning, measures bodies electrical activity of seven energy centers, result obtain in the form of number & coloured bar graphs. First SSRF noted original reading of energy, then they offered veg food to few peoples and non-veg food to few peoples, after this consecutive readings are taken after 1 to 4 hours interval, **peoples who taken veg food shown positive improvement in energy and those who consumed non veg food shown fall in their energy.**

Reference chart for various food types

SATTVIC	RAJAS	TAMASIC
Food Which Give Goodness or Purity of Thoughts	Food which gives Bad emotions	Food Which Gives Dullness or inertia
Cow's milk	Fish	Beef
Cream	Eggs	Pork
Cheese	Meat	Wine
Butter	Salt	Onions
Curd	Chilies	Garlic
Ghee	Chutney	Tobacco
Sweet fruits	Asafoetida	Rotten things
Apples	Pickles	Stale things
Bananas	Tamarind	Unclean things
Grapes	Mustard	Twice cooked things
Pomegranates	Hot things	All liquors
Mangoes	Tea	All drugs
Oranges	Coffee	
Pears	Cocoa	
Pineapples	Ovaltine	
Guavas	White sugar	
Figs	Carrots	
Vegetables	Turnips	
Coconut	Spices	
Brinjals		
Potatoes		
Cabbages		
Spinach		

DO & DON'TS OF BATH AS PER AYURVEDA

This article in not applicable for cold areas where snowfall occurs. It is applicable for normal areas.

Benefits of Cold Water Bath

Water should be of room temperature.

1. It helps in getting rid of laziness.
2. It tends to stimulate nerve endings & gives a fresh start in morning.
3. It increases release of the depression beating chemicals like beta endorphins. And thus help to get out of depression.
4. Studies show that it helps to improve reproductive health in men by stimulating release of testosterone.
5. It also helps in improving lungs function.
6. Cold water bath stimulates the lymphatic & immune system of the body, there by boosting production of cells that fight against infections.

Benefits of Warm Water Bath

Water temperature can be slightly above room temperature.

1. Warm temperature tend to kill the germs more. So it cleanses the body.
2. It is useful for unhealthy persons, for example person suffering with high temperature.
3. It improves flexibility of muscles, and also helps relax sore muscles.
4. It reduces sugar levels in body, so making your body less prone to diabetes.
5. It is beneficial to treat cough and cold.

Ayurvedic Guildelines on Bath

1. For youngsters it is suggested to bath with cold water & for old peoples it is suggested to bath with hot water.
2. For students who are dedicated to studies, cold water bath will be beneficial.
3. If your body type is PITTA (warm hands),it is better to have cold water bath.
4. If your body type is KAPHA/VATA (cold hands), it is better to have hot water bath.
5. If you work out regularly, warm water bath is suggested.
6. If you bath in morning it is better to have cold water bath, if you are taking bath at night, it is better to have warm water bath. As evening time is dominated by VATA.

Do's & don't's

- Avoid hot water pouring on head & eyes. As per Ayurveda it is place of KAPHA. It can increase KAPHA & related diseases.
- Eyes must be cleaned with cold water only. While cleaning eyes, cold water should be kept in mouth.
- For body pain & muscles pain, alternate warm & cold water can be poured on affected area. It will relax those muscles.
- If you don't bath daily, it reduces your productivity. So it is must to bath daily.
- Instead of chemical soaps, prepare paste of following and use. You can try different combination as below. And rub on your body. It will clear all holes on your skin.
  Milk & multi grain flour.
  Milk & split Bengal gram.
  Milk & Turmeric powder.
  Water & neem tree leaves
  Water & rose flower leaves
- Bath should be ended with normal cold water.
- If you are bathing with cold water, start it from head.
- If you are bathing with warm water, start it from legs.

- Never eat before bath, bath will stop your digestion.
- Never swim after eating.
- After bath rub your body with towel. It will help to clear holes on your skin.
- Never have multiple baths in day, it will reduce your energy.
- After bath put one or two drops of mustered oil in naval region. It will give you glow on face.

ALKALINE FOOD CAN SAVE FROM 46 TO 50 DISEASES

If acidic forming food is replaced with alkaline forming food, then it can improve health. Foods whatever we eat can change acidity or alkalinity of body (the pH value).

When we metabolize foods and extract the energy (calories) from them, we are actually burning the foods, except that it happens in a slow and controlled fashion. When we burn foods, they actually leave an ash residue, just like when we burn wood in a furnace. As it turns out, this ash can be acidic or alkaline (or neutral),and proponents of this diet claim that this ash can directly affect the acidity of our body.

So if we eat foods with acidic ash, it makes our body acidic. If we eat foods with alkaline ash, it makes our body alkaline. Neutral ash has no effect.

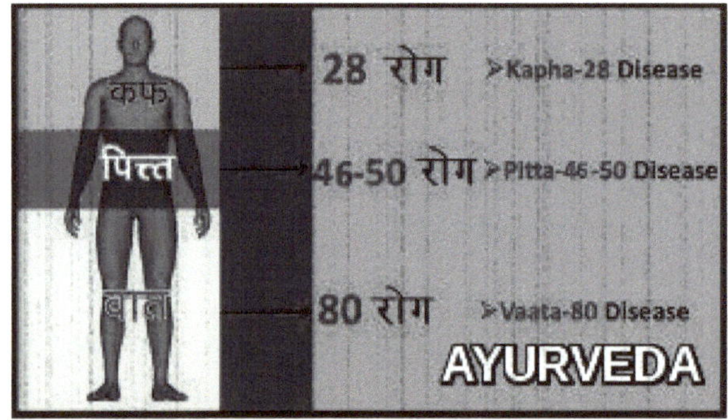

Acid ash is thought to make us vulnerable to illness and disease, whereas alkaline ash is considered protective. By choosing more alkaline foods, we should be able to alkalize our diet and improve our health.

Food components that leave an acidic ash include protein, phosphate and sulfur, while alkaline components include calcium, magnesium, and potassium.

When talking about the alkaline diet, it is important to understand the meaning of the pH value. Put simply, the pH value is a measure of how acidic or alkaline something is.

- ✓ The pH value ranges from 0 to 14:
- ✓ 0-7 is acidic.
- ✓ 7 is neutral.
- ✓ 7–14 is alkaline (alkaline is often called basic).

Many proponents of this diet suggest that people monitor the pH value of their urine using test strips, making sure that it is alkaline (pH over 7) and not acidic (below 7).

It is important to note that pH value has variation in our body at different components of the body.

The stomach is loaded with hydrochloric acid, giving it a pH value between 2 and 3.5 (highly acidic). This is necessary to break down food.

On the other hand, human blood is always slightly alkaline, with a pH between 7.35 and 7.45.

Food Affects the pH of our Urine, But Not our Blood

It is critical for health that the pH of our blood remains constant. If it goes out of the normal range, our cells would stop working and we would die very quickly if left untreated. For this reasons our body has its own mechanism to maintain pH value of our blood.

However, food can definitely change the pH value of the urine. This is actually one of the main ways our body regulates blood pH... by excreting acids in our urine.

This indicates that Alkaline food can save us from kidney disease. And also saves us from acidity problem, which can create many diseases in our stomach, lever & large intestine.

Many alkaline diet enthusiasts believe that in order to maintain a constant blood pH, the body takes alkaline minerals (such as calcium) from your bones to buffer the acids from the acid-forming foods you eat. But it is yet to be proved scientifically.

HOME REMEDY OF CONSTIPATION

Triphala Churn(powder) is made from following three fruits, all these three are ayurvedic shrubs found in INDIA

1. Amla (Indian gooseberry)
2. Baheda (Terminalia bellirica)
3. Harad (Terminalia chebula)

Ratio for making Triphala Churna is as below
 Amla 300 grams + Baheda 200 grams + Harad 100 grams

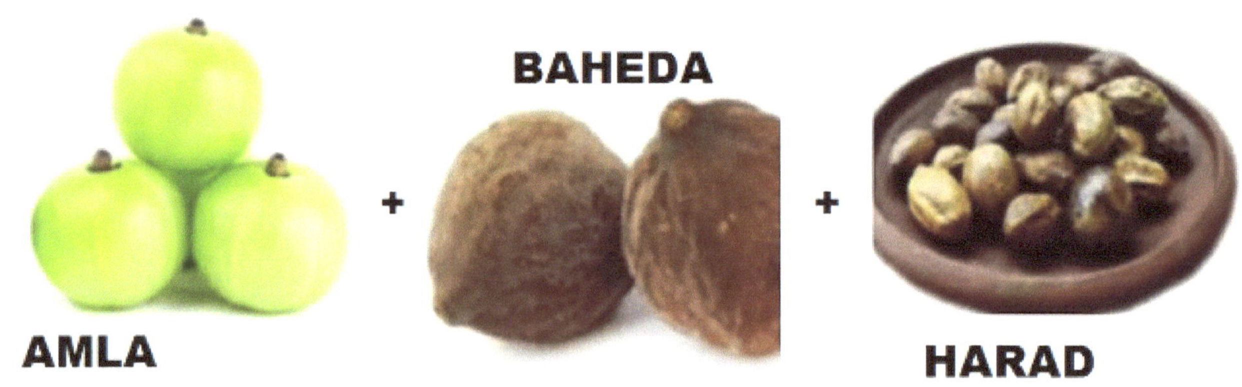

It can make a balance of Vata, Pitta (Acidty) & cough. If this balance is maintained in our body, you will not have any disease.

Method for usage

Before sleeping, you have to mix one spoon of triphala churn with one glass of water. In morning you will find that it cleans your stomach.

If Some peoples found that it has less effect, next day you can increase its quantity two spoons. But never use more than two spoons.

Regular use will remove constipation; it can remove old constipation of even 30 to 40 years. After using it for three months, you have to take a break of 15 days, so that our body should not get habitual of this. It do not have any side effects.

In morning after getting fresh you can take it with honey or jaggery, then it will act as vitamin supplement for body. It contains all necessary vitamins & micro nutrients.

If any person gets harmful radiation attack, then he can take Triphala churn with equal ratio of all three fruits. It can give him fast recovery from illness.

As per scientific research Amla has very high anti-oxidant properties. Due to oxidation ageing increases, it reduces efficiency of body parts. With regular consumption of Amla, you can retain youth & remain fit and energetic. With regular usage of Amla, you can reduce weight.

Top reason for constipation

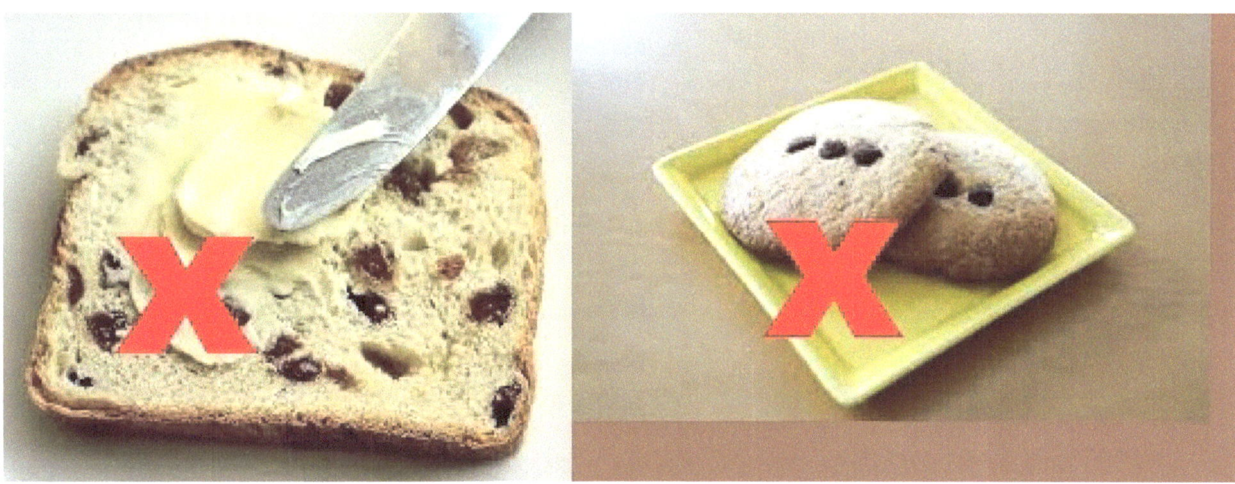

Never eat bakery items made from Maida like bread and biscuits.
Maida has adhesive property, which can lead to blockage of large intestine.
Maida is a wheat flour from the Indian subcontinent. Finely milled without any bran, refined, and bleached, it closely resembles Cake flour. The term maida is common in southern India; the equivalent term in northern India is safed atta, literally "white flour", though maida is also very common in the north.

THE NATURAL FOODS FOR ANTI AGEING

Your looks have lot of importance, so you must look young and energetic. Whatever food we are discussing here, it will make you young & glow of your skin will also increase by around 10 times. With this food your ageing process will become slow.

With regular usage of these foods, a 35 year old man can look like a 20 year old boy. And 50 year old man can look young as of 35 year.

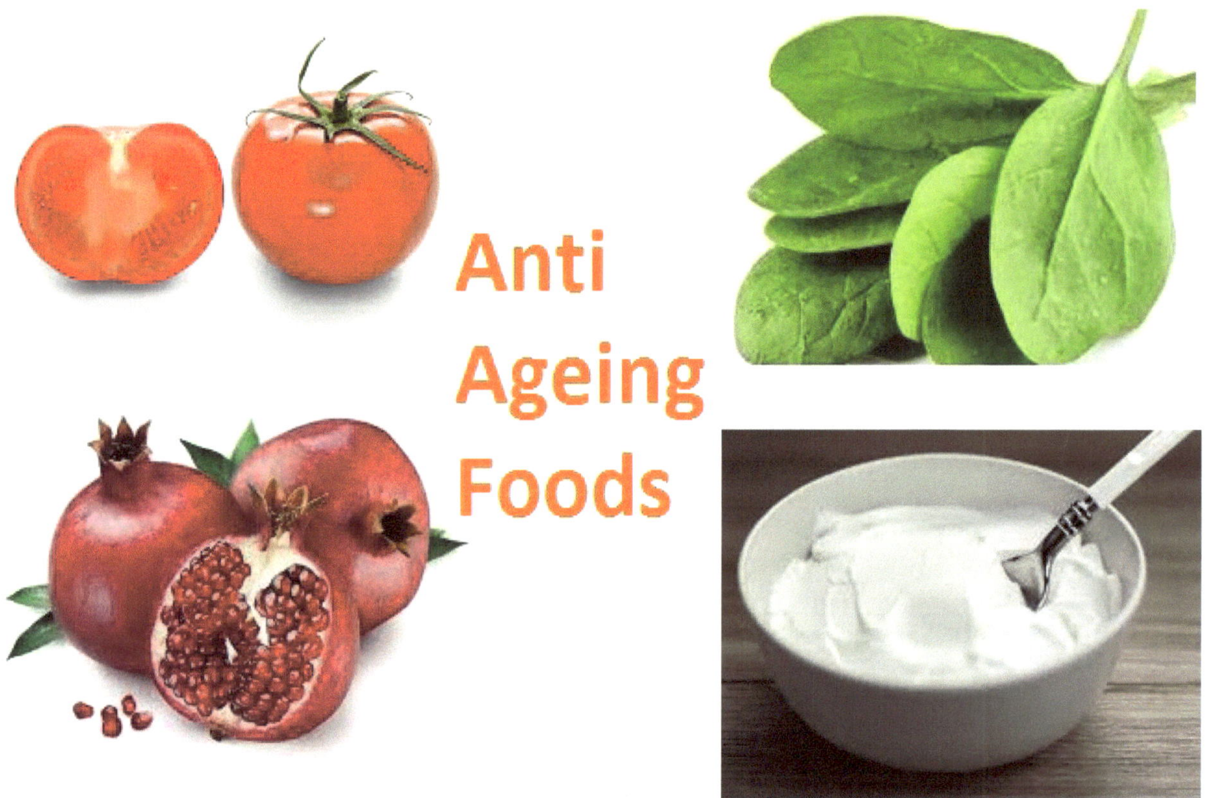

These foods are as below.

Yogurt

It is a rich source of protein and calcium. Protein strengthen your muscles & calcium gives strength to your bones. Yogurt contains millions of bacteria, which strengthen your digestive system. Most of disease comes due to improper digestion. But if your digestion system is strong, it will maintain your health.

Carrot

It keeps your eyes healthy. It helps to remove any eye disease.It improves night vision. It is also helpful for health of your teeth. It helps to recover from any disease related to teeth. It gives you glowing skin. If you are regularly eating carrot , then it increase your brain power, it helps to understand any critical subjects.

Pomegranate

It contains large amount of vitamin C, it help to guard skin against wrinkling effect caused by sun. It contains both ellagic acid and punicalagin. The fist fight with free radicals & second is super nutrient, it can increase body capacity to preserve collagen, the sub dermal connective tissue that makes skin looks smooth and plump.

Orange

It is rich source of vitamin C, it also contains potassium and magnesium. It helps to control blood pressure.

It improves your blood circulation. So it is helpful for all body organs. It keeps your heart healthy. It reduces skin problems like wrinkles & pimples

Tomato

It contains vitamin A and vitamin C. Both these vitamins gives you glowing skin. Vitamin A is very good for eyes, it improves vision. In market lot of anti ageing creams are available, these creams contains tomato juice in large amount. Which is mixed with various other chemicals. So regular usage of tomato will keep your skin glowing and healthy.

Spinach leaves

It is better than all above. It is a very healthy food on this planet. It contains vitamin K. It also contains zinc and magnesium. It reduces hypertension. It is also very good for healthy eyes. It also gives strength to your bones. It gives your better sleep. It improves your immune system. It reduces pimples. It also improves interconnectivity of neurons, due to which memory power & brain processing speed also improves.

Your skin wrinkles comes due to free radicals. Spinach removes these free radicals. That is why your skin starts glowing.

Only looking young is not sufficient, it should also be coordinated with a strong and powerful brain. Spinach helps to achieve both these things.

So include these foods in your regular diet & remain young and healthy.

INDIAN EATING HABITS AS PER AYURVEDA

1. Food should be chewed slowly. Chew as many times, which is equal to no. of teeth's. If a person has 28 teeth's, then he should chew food for 28 times. If a person has 32 teeth's, then he should chew for 32 times.

2. Before eating mind & body must be stress free & relaxed, that is why in India, before eating we pray & chant some Mantra. It gives relaxation of mind.

3. Drink water which is stored in earthen pot, it gives necessary minerals for body. Never use cold water from refrigerator.

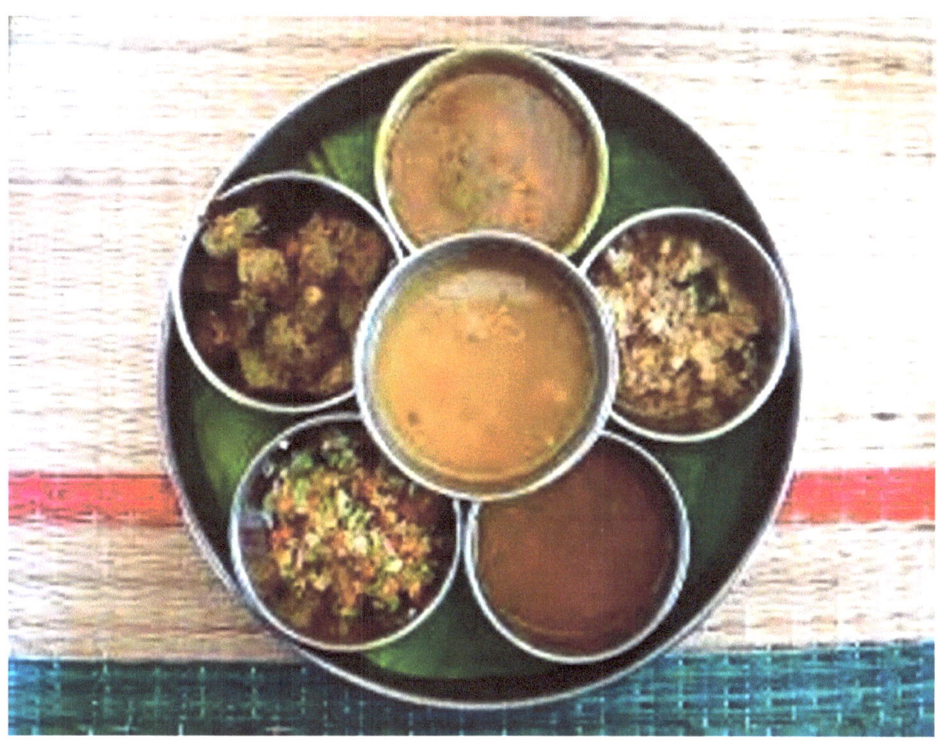

4. Try to sit in Indian style on floor, it keeps your center of gravity at your naval point, it helps in better digestion of food. Now peoples have got habit of dining table. Please observe your comfort in both conditions siting on chair & siting on floor, after continuous observation you will be convinced that by siting on floor, you will be more relaxed & digestion is better.

5. In night drinking water should be kept in copper pot, after awakening in morning, this water should be sipped, it reduces acidity.

6. After eating a small piece of jaggery around 20 to 25 grams, should be chewed, it is alkaline in nature, it reduces acidity. Good for digestion.

7. Never eat twice cooked food.

8. Cooked food is best for eating within 45 minutes to 1 hour only, after cooking.

9. Wheat, Jawar, Grams(Dal) powder is best for 7 days to 15 days only, after grinding.

10. Morning meal should be taken within 2.5 hours of sunrise, in this period digestive system is more active. Digestive enzymes are related to power of sunlight.

11. Concept of a little breakfast is better suited in those countries where there is a snow fall & peoples are unable to see regular sunrise. In India we can see daily sunrise, so system of little breakfast is not suitable.

12. In morning you can take heavy food & also try different test. In afternoon reduce food by on third & in evening again reduce food by on third.

13. Evening Dinner should be done before sunset. Before sleeping our food gets digested, so we can get good sleep. Veg food generally requires 10 to 12 hours for full digestion. So before sunrise on next morning ,our stomach can get empty. We can get a good start of day.

14. Eating for three times is suggested only for those who are doing physical work. Those who are working in office and do not have physical activity, for them eating only twice in sufficient.

15. All these habits will give you good health. It will reduce diabetes, bad cholesterol, will reduce fat etc.

HEALTH BENEFITS OF GOMUTRA (COW'S URINE)

As per Maharishi Vagbhatta cow is the most admirable gift given by god to mankind. He does lot of appreciation of Gomutra (Cows's Urine). Gomutra do not have any side effects.

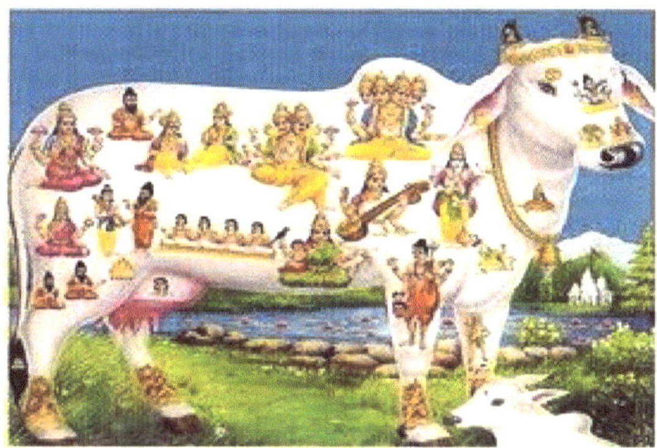

It contains 95% water. Despite of water it contains calcium, sulpher, iron, siliocon, boron, manganese, magenesium,curcumin etc. Like this gomutra contains 18 micro nutrients. Which are very necessary for human body. All these micro nutrients are in digestible form.

It is used for following disease.

Diabetes, cancer, arthritis, bronchitis, bronchial pneumonia, eye disease like ratinal detachment & gluocoma, crack heels, hair disease, Tuberculosis, all types of skin diseases etc.

How to take Gomutra

- It should be drinked in early morning with empty stomach.
- Persons having some disease, should take 100 ml in one day. It can be divided in two parts 50 ml in morning & 50 ml in evening.
- Healthy peoples if want to take to maintain immunity and health, they should take 50 ml in morning only.
- Gomutra must be fresh,then only it will give results. If gomutra is stored for few days, then its micro nutrients reduces as per time.

- Cow must be Of Indian origin. They have bump on their back.

Gomutra Limitations

- It can alone give complete relief from vata & kapha diseases.
- But for pitta (acidity), some minor medicines are added to gomutra as per suggestion of expert doctors in Ayurveda.
- Patients of acidity, should dilute gomutra with water, suppose you are taking 50 ml of gomutra then add 100 ml of water in it.
- Ladies should not take gomutra during period of mensuration cycle. For rest of the period they can take.
- Cows which are peged, their gomutra is of no use, cow must have daily sufficient walking & must be healthy.
- Cows which have delivered calfs in last three- four months, they are giving milk regularly. So their gomutra has less micro ingredients.

- Cow should not be pregnant, she should be healthy. Gomutra of cow calf should be preferred. Calf's are young, energetic & always wonder here & there. So their gomutra conins 18 micro nutrients. Which are necessary for human body.

Skin Disease

Skin diseas occuer due to low sulpher in body. In this case daily gomutra is suggested to drink by patient. Also it can be applied on affected skin area .

Gomutra is very helpful is recovery from psoriasis, you need to apply Gomutra on affected areas & do massage with your hands.It can cure any skin disease including itching.

Regular usage can give result in 45 to 60 days.

Joint pen

It is very helpful in recovery of all type of joint pain like knee pain, lumber pain, shoulder pain etc. Regular usage can give relief in 15 to 30 days.

Tuberculosis (TB)

It is very helpful in recovery from TB. Government recommends Dots tablets for TB, with this tablets patient need 6 to 8 months for recovery. But if Gomutra is regulary used along with dots. It can give relief in 45 to 60 days only .The patient who used gomutra will never get back TB. Because gomuti increase immunity & resistance power of body. It is tested by Honorable Bhai Rajiv Dixit in AIIMS (All India Institute of Medical Sciences)

Cough & Cold

Any disease caused by kapha imbalance like cough and cold, can be easily cured with usage of Gomutra.

Cancer

Due to use of tobacco products, some people's gets abscess in mouth, which is first stage of cancer, take gomutra in mouth, keep for few minutes & rinse it & throw out, it will give recovery from abscess.

Main reason of cancer is lack of curcumin in body. Gomutra contains good amount of curcumin,it is in digestable form. So it is very useful is cancer treatment. Thus Gomutra can cure Throat Cancer, Esophagus cancer & Intestine cancer. For other types of cancers, research is going on at "Valsad Ayrvedic Cancer Hospital" which located in Gujrat state.

Cow should be respected & kept for Gomutra. Milk is secondary benefit which is available for a limited period but gomutra is available for lifetime of the cow.

For Hair fall & dandruff

Put some gomutra in water, and do massage of your head with this. Wash out after 10 minutes. With regular usage it will give relief from hair diseases.

HOME REMEDY OF CRACK HEELS

First Method

Take one yellow colored banana & cut into small pieces and make its paste by grinding. Rub this paste on your feet's. Allow to dry it for 15 to 20 minutes. Then wash it with warm water. Do this three times a week. With regular usage, It will recover your cracks.

Second Method

Take two spoons of milk cream & add one spoon of lemon juice in it. Rub this mixture on feet's before sleeping. In morning after wake up wash your feet's with warm water, it will recover cracks on feet's. Use it daily till recovery.

I have tested it successfully for grand mother, she has got fast recovery of cracks. With creams suggested by skin specialist doctors, she doesn't get any benefit, but this Ayurveda home remedy has given good results.

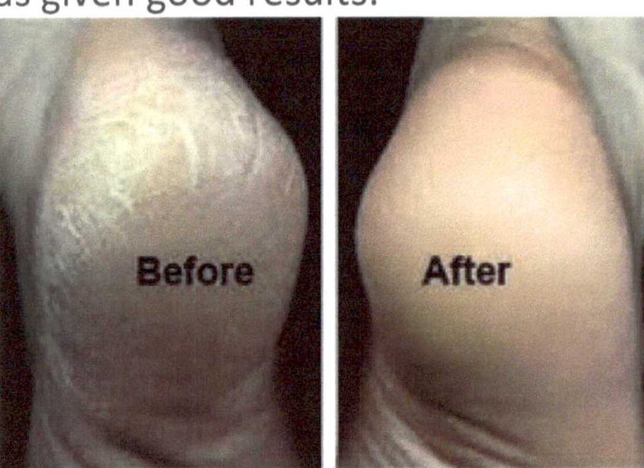

Third Method

Take one spoon of petroleum jelly & add one spoon lemon juice. Make a good mixture. Apply this on cracks before sleeping. Wear socks on it. In morning wash feet's with warm water. It can be used on every alternate day till recovery.

NATURAL REMEDY OF STOMACH GAS

It is a very common problem with most of the peoples, especially for aged persons. It can make them a butt of ridicule.

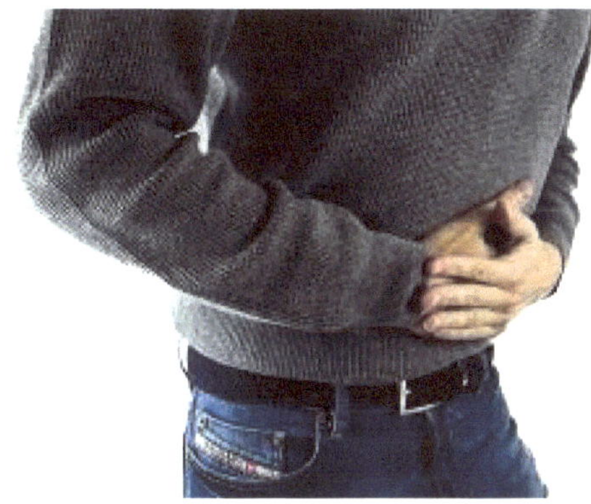

Top reasons of gas formation.

1. Improper digestion and old age.
2. Tea and coffee creates gases.
3. Alcohal, bear, smoking etc. also causes gas formation.
4. Eating fast without proper chewing.
5. If your stomach remain empty for a long time, it can lead to acidity & gas formation.
6. More spicy food, Junk food, fried up food etc.
7. Overeating
8. Taking cold drink with meal.
9. Cabbage , Chana Dal, Potato, Udad dal, Rajma etc.
10. Drinking water with meal or immediately after meal, leads to improper digestion.

Home remedy for Gases

1. If you eat on clove and a cardamom after meal, it helps to prevents gas formation and acidity also.
2. If you utilize Ajwain as spices in food, it helps in digestion process and prevents gas formation.
3. Take two buds of Garlic, cut into small pieces, and swallow with one glass of warm water in morning with empty stomach.
4. Lemon tea (Without any milk), helps to reduce gas formation.

5. Take one spoon of rock salt with one glass of warm water in morning with empty stomach.
6. Alo vera juice with triphala (Ayurved medicine in India) powder helps to prevent gas formation.
7. Lemon juice two spoons, add some rock salt & take with one glass of warm water. It reduces gas formation.
8. Methi (Fenugreek) tea made with water, reduces gas formation. But it can cause increase in acidity.
9. Take half spoon cinnamon powder, boil with water, after cooling mix half spoon honey, take this mixture with empty stomach in morning. It also prevents gas formation.

Most helpful remedy

1. Take a small piece of ginger, after that take a glass of warm water, it prevents gas formation.
2. Take a spoon of jeera powder , mix with cold water. You have to take this after meal. It helps in digestion and prevent gas formation.
3. Take a small piece of Jaggery, after meal. It helps digestion & prevents gas formation.

Ayurvedic medicine for gas

Divya Gas Har Chunrna by Patnjali (Ramdev Baba's Product)

HEALTH BENEFITS FENUGREEK SEEDS (METHI SEEDS)

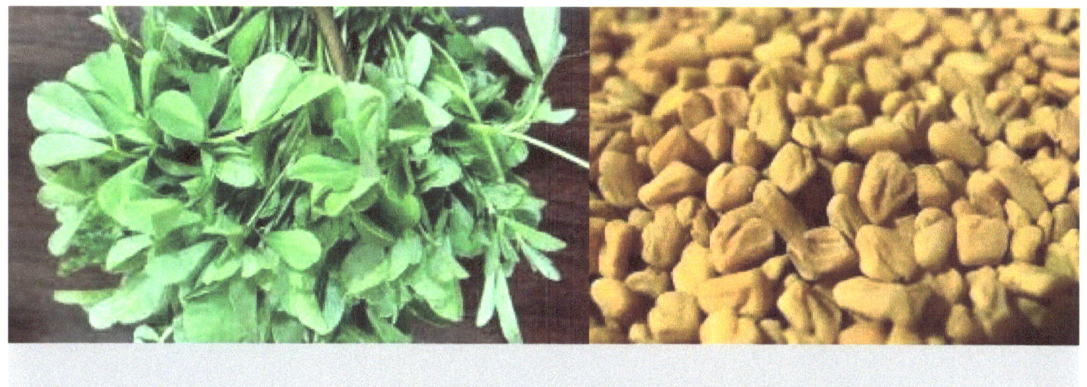

Methi contains good amount of iron, phosphorus, magnesium, manganese, copper etc. It also contains vitamin B-6,It is antioxidant, antiviral, anti-inflammatory .It do not have any side effects & it do not have any expiry date also. Methi seeds are used as spices to enhance taste & smell of food. If you eat methi seeds daily morning, it help to reduce obesity. It is also helpful for growth of breast.

It is having high electromagnetic force as compared to any other drugs & foods. If you have any pain in the body, put 4 to 5 methi seeds on that place, put cello tape on that, after few minutes you will find that pain is removed from body.

How to Make Methi Laddu (Sweet Meat)

Take powder of methi seeds, mix with cow's ghee & jaggery (Gul/GUD-HINDI word) & make its laddu. These are very useful for protection from cold. And all other diseases mentioned below.

How to Make Methi Tea

Take around 2 cup of water, mix 1 spoon of methi seeds & boil it, then filter it. You can mix honey for sweet taste as per your choice. After cooling down you can sip it.

Diabetes

Methi seeds (Fenugreek seeds) is very useful in diabetes, you have to put 1 spoon (around 10 to 12 grams) in one glass of water in evening, allow it to soak for whole night, in morning after awakening, you have to drink this water after that you have to chew this methi seeds.

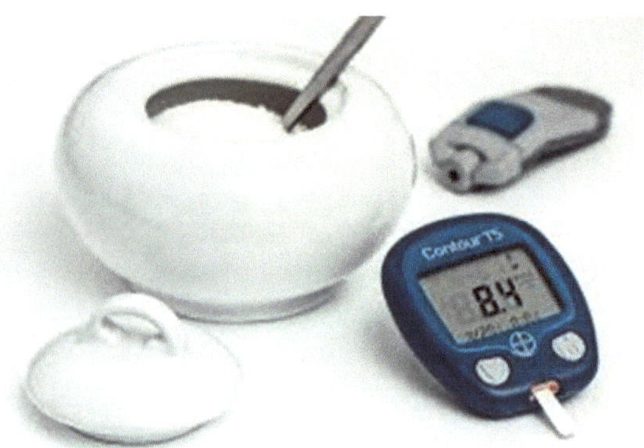

 If anybody does this regularly for three months, he will be totally relived from diabetes. After this do not eat or drink anything for one hour. Normal person without any disease can take this for two weeks, after 2 weeks, take interval of 2 weeks, after that same sequence can be continued. It is also useful in hypertension.

For cold

A Methi seed contains good antioxidant properties. So it helps in recovery from flue and cold. It also have antibacterial & antiviral properties.

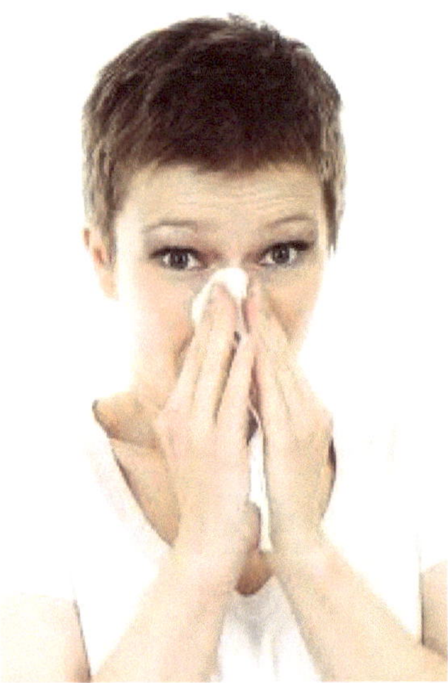

 So helpful in fighting with harmful bacteria and virus. You can eat daily one laddu (sweet meat) for recovery. For faster recovery you can drink methi tea for 2 to 3 times a day. To reduce throat sensation, you can do gargling with methi tea.

Female reproductive system

It is especially useful for ladies who undergone seaserian operation far faster recovery. Those who eat this laddu (Sweetmeat) during pregnancy, then chance of seaserian delivery are equal to none. It is good source of galatcagogues, it improves milk formation in breast.

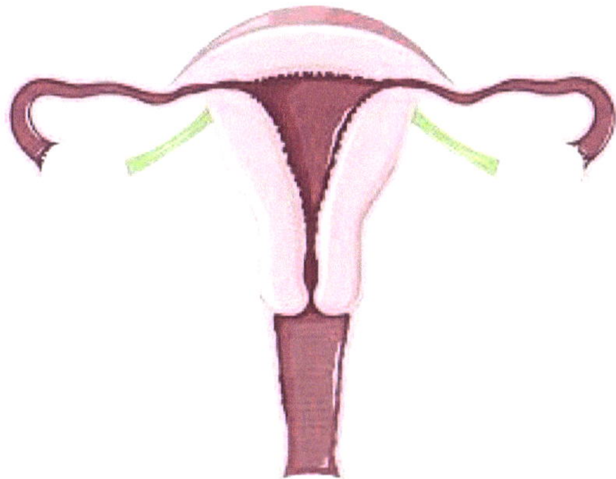

It contains vitamins and magnesium, which improved quality of milk also.It is very useful in the case of uterus displacement for faster recovery. Eating daily one Laddu for around 3 months will ensure uterus is back in place. Methi seeds are reach source of iron, so it stimulates formation of red blood cells. So it helps in blood recovery. Any disease related to mensuration cycle can be cured with this. It is also very helpful in menopause, it restores hormonal balance.

Heart disease

It is also very useful in reducing bad cholesterol (LDL). Cholesterol is root cause of coronary artery disease, which can lead to heart attack.

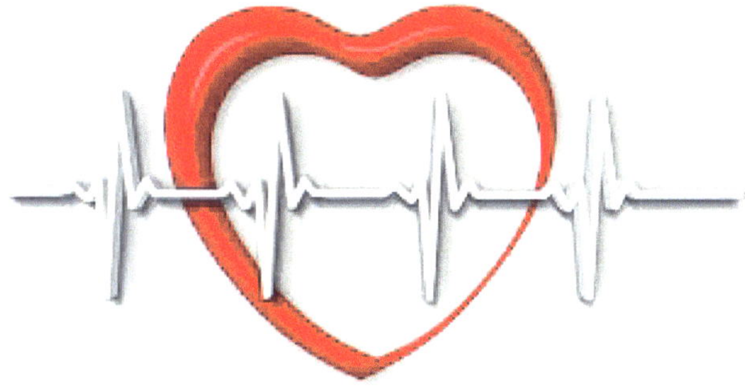

To reduce risk of heart attack, you can drink tea of Methi seeds daily. Also you can eat one Laddu (Sweet meat) daily.

For Ear Pain in children's

Boil methi funds in coconut oil/cow ghee/mustered oil, allow it to cool down, one or two drops of these oil can be poured in ear. It will relive the child from ear pain.

For Dog Bite

You can make paste of methi powder & water. You can put this paste on that place, is very helpful for fast recovery.

For Constipation

Methi seeds are good source of soluble fibers. In evening take one spoon methi seeds powder, mix with water and drink at the time of sleeping. Regular usage will remove constipation. It is also helpful for good sleep. It increases hunger & digestion. Is also helpful in stomach pain. It also reduces acidity.

For Facial beauty.

Its anti-oxidant properties save you from free radical damage of skin. It also make your face beautiful.

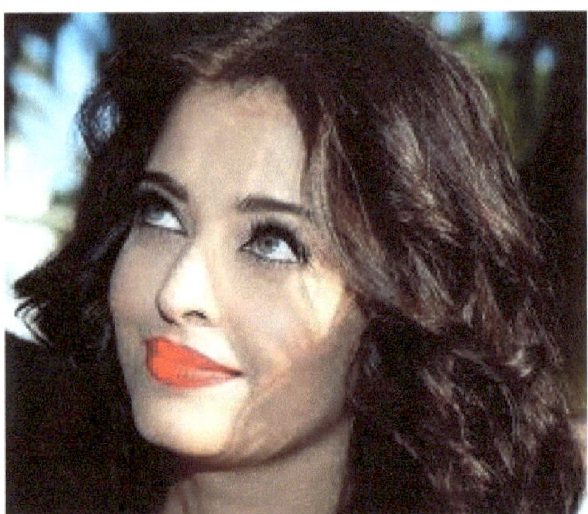

You have to apply paste of seeds mixed with curds, apply for half an hour & then scrub with your hands & wash face with cold water, it removed dead cells, & give you a fresh glowing look. It is also useful in hair diseases.

Arthritis (Vat diseases)

It is also very helpful in Vat diseases for example Knee joint pen, shoulder pain, ankle pain etc. A Methi seed contains iron, calcium & phosphorus, which are helpful for bones. Its anti-inflammatory properties reduce joint swelling.

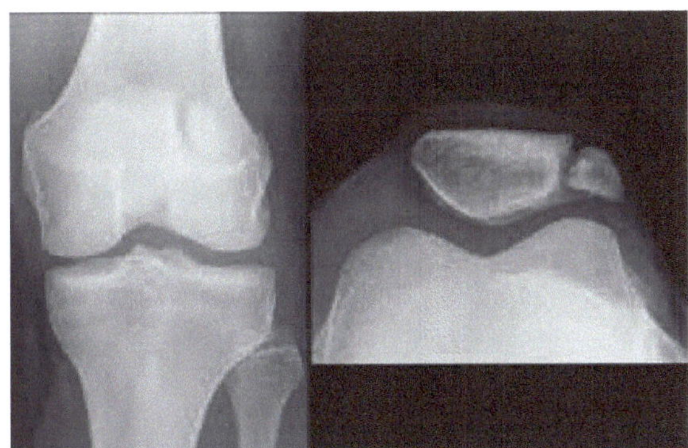

 For joint pain you can apply paste of methi seeds powder mixed with water, on joint. After drying this paste, you can wash it with warm water. You can repeat this procedure for two to three times, till you get relief from pain.

Methi Seed's Precautions.

1. Excessive usage can result in diarrhea.
2. Before using you can do taste for checking allergy. Put some powder on your skin and check for its effect.
3. If you are taking any medical treatment, then before taking methi seeds consult your doctor/physician.

NEVER EAT INCOMPATIBLE FOODS.

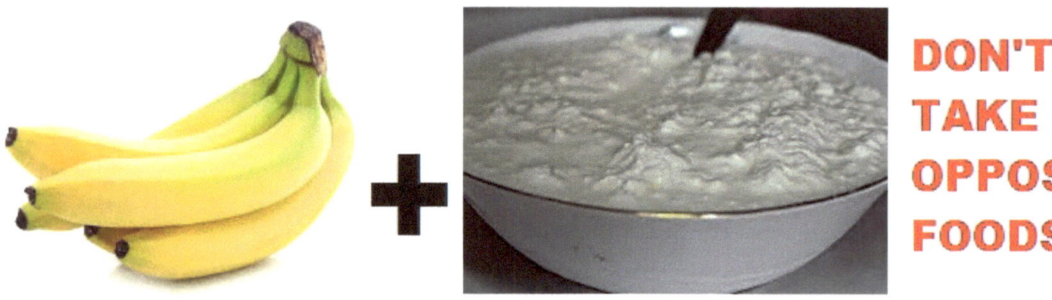

1. Curds & udad dal—increases hypertension
2. Curds & banana
3. Curds & non veg
4. Curds & tomato
5. Curds & tomato—increase kapha in respiratory system
6. Curds is not allowed in dinner- slow down digestion
7. Tea & biscuits
8. Tea & citrus fruits
9. Tomoato & ker
10. Milk & salty food
11. milk & jack fruit

12. Milk & mango (having citric acid)
13. Milk & fruits having citric acid (pterocarpus)
14. milk & onion---- -creates skin disease

15. Milk & other animal prodcuts (egg & non veg, honey etc.)
16. Milk & brinjal
17. milk & muli (vegetable again)
18. Milk & banana
19. Never keep ghee in copper pots
20. Beer & salty foods-----increases salt in our blood
21. Carrot & lemon-------causes heart burn & urine related problems
22. Honey & grapes
23. Honey & muli (vegetable again)

24.Honey & ghee
25.Non veg & potato
26.Non veg & milk
27.Non veg & curds
28.Non veg & sprouts
29.Non veg & cheese
30.Non veg & roti/chapati made with maida
31.Fish & eags
32.Non veg should not be cooked in teel (by) oil.

Potato & Maida contains starch in it, for its digestion; body needs more alkaline juice, on other hand non veg contains protein, for digestion of protein body needs more acid. So such mixture do not digest properly, it creates harmful gases & decay of food.

Maida is a wheat flour from the Indian subcontinent. Finely milled without any bran, refined, and bleached, it closely resembles Cake flour. The term maida is common in southern India; the equivalent term in northern India is safed atta, literally "white flour", though maida is also very common in the north.

HEALTH BENEFITS OF TURMERIC

It is very useful and has lot of heath benefits. It is useful from recovery from cough and cold.

It can cure any throat disease .It is also useful for treatment of tonsils. It is anti-bacterial, anti-fungal & anti-viral, so it makes our immune system strong.

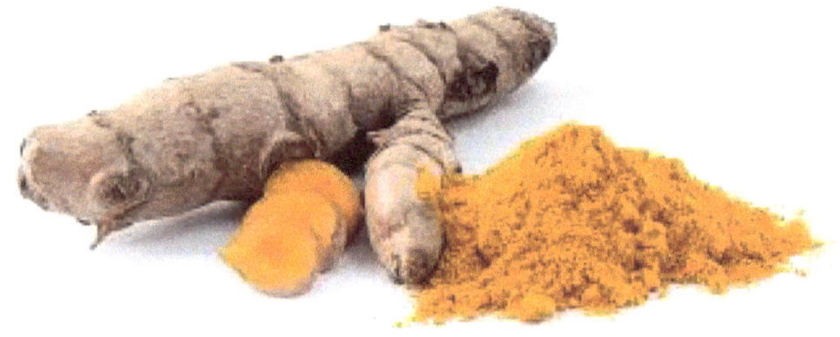

How to take turmeric

Turmeric powder can be mixed with either warm water or warm milk & then sip slowly. It can be also taken with by mixing with honey of cow's ghee. In a cup of milk 5 to 10 grams of turmeric can be taken at one time.

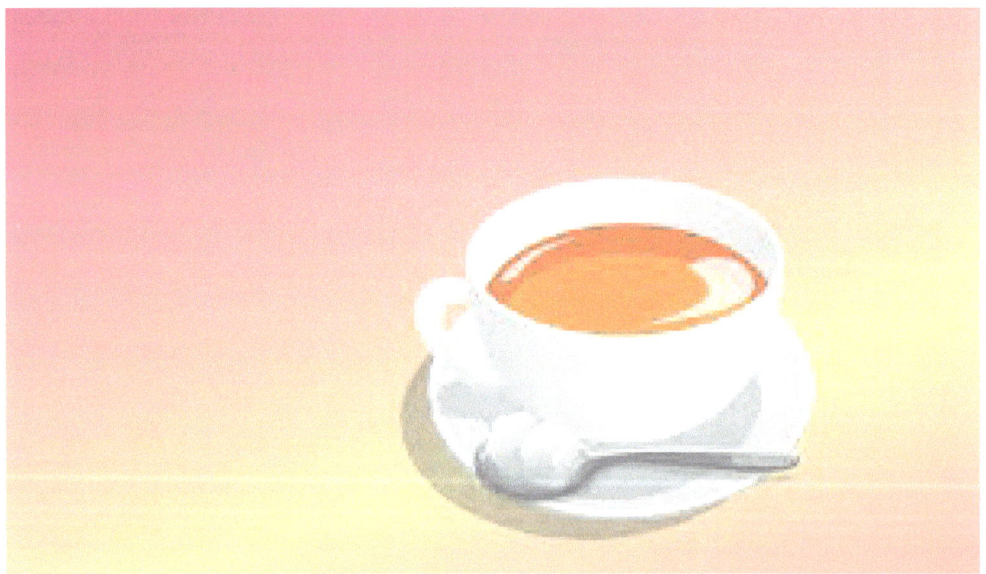

Tonsils treatment

For tonsil treatment, you can put 5 to 10 grams of dry powder in throat. In next 5 to 7 minutes, it will mix with saliva & will go down to stomach. After doing this for 2 to 3 times in a week, children's will be relived from tonsil problems.

Other benefits

Turmeric is also helpful for purification of blood. If blood is purified, generally no diseases will occurs. It has antiviral, antibiotic and anti-inflammatory properties.

If you get some minor injury, put dry turmeric powder on it, it will help in fast recovery. It is also very useful for improvement of skin colors. If you want become white from black, you have take daily turmeric-milk regularly for long duration. It is hundred times better than cosmetic creams.

Peoples, who are suffering from sun burn or sun stroke, can put directly dry powder on their skin. It is also helpful for continence (Brmahacharya).

Cancer Treatment

It is very useful for cancer treatment, it contain one element curcumin, which is the main element for cancer treatment. It is found mainly in INDIAN turmeric Fresh turmeric which is brought from farms, its juice contains curcumin. This juice can be mixed with honey

Remedy of lever disease

Turmeric is also useful in liver diseases, it increase enzymes which are helpful in removing toxic substances from liver.

For glowing skin

Make a paste of milk & turmeric powder, use on your face, after drying scrub with your hands & then wash your face with cold water, it helps to removes black stains and dead skin & also gives glow to your skin.

Remove unwanted hairs.

If you want to remove unwanted hairs, make a paste of warm coconut oil & turmeric powder. Now apply this cream on unwanted hairs. Regular usage will remove these hairs slowly & will also make the skin soft.

Remedy of Stomach disease

Turmeric is used as spices in making food. Correct usage helps to reduce acidity & alsar formation as well as recovery.

Remedy of Teeth Ache

Make a paste of Turmeric powder, salt & mustered oil. With this massage on roots of tooth, It reduces inflation and bacteria.

Precaution of Turmeric

1. Persons having gall bladder stone should not take turmeric
2. It reduces sperm activity
3. Diabetic persons should not take turmeric.
4. Peoples who are suffering with less iron should not take turmeric.
5. If yoh have a planned surgery are recently undergone surgery, then do not take turmeric, as it can slow down blood clotting.

HEALTH BENEFITS OF TULSI (HOLY BASIL) पवित्र तुलसी

Tulsi is treated as goddess of HINDU'S. Tulsi is used in Pooja (Prayer of god) except Ganesha & Shiva. Tulsi leafs should be never chewed, instead of it can be swallowed. If we chew tulsi leafs, it will be harmful for our teeth's. Dried plant of tulsi should be never kept in house, it can be thrown in flowing rivers. Instead of it plant a new fresh tulsi. Tulsi removes negative energy from our house. Never pluch tulsi leafs in night, Sundays,sun & moon grahan kal. It is treated as very harmful. Tulsi leafs can be used upto 12 days after plucking, for Pooja (Rituals), water can be showered on it, & it can be used in rituals. In evening times, Lamp should be ignited in front of Tusli. It will give blessings of Mahalaxmi (Goddess of wealth).Tulsi emits ozone (O3), so it keeps atmosphere fresh and healthy. Tulsi saves us from lot of diseases. Tulsi leafs can not be plucked without bath, otherwise at the time of rituals Gods do not accept such leafs.

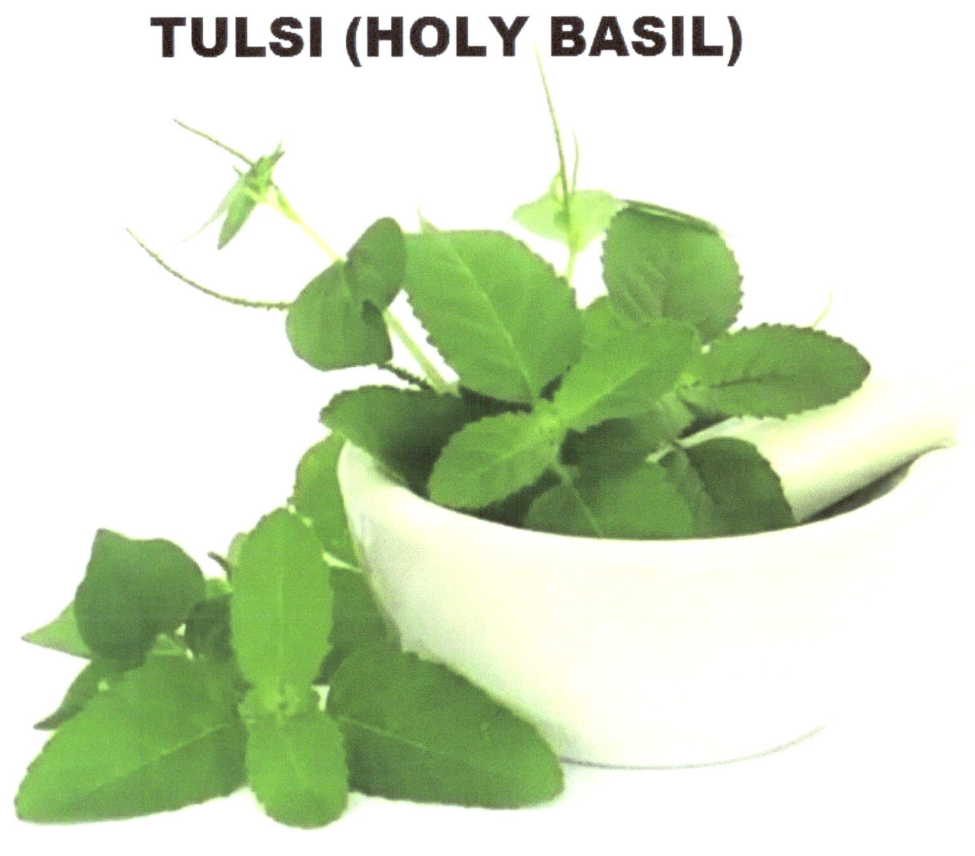

Medical Use

Tulsi has antioxidant properties, it works as anti bacterial, anti fungal & anti biotic agent for our body. Healthy person can eat daily 4 to 5 leafs. For treatment of some disease, 4 to 5 leafs can be taken twice, once in morning and once in evening. Tulsi can give relief from stress. It purifies our blood. It improves our immunity. It gives glow to our skin.

For Loose Motion

If you have loose motions, take some tulsi leafs, grind it, add some honey and Jeera powder. This mixture will give relief from loose motion.

For Omitting

For Omitting, add some ginger juice in tulsi juice, this mixture will give relief.

For Cancer

Tulsi leafs are also helpful in fighting cancer, if you are swallowing few tulsi leafs daily, then it prevents growth of cancer cells in our body.

For Temperature

If you are suffering with temperature, it may be due to malaria or viral infection. Tulsi kadha (Mixture of tulsi with other elements) can give relief.

How to Make Tulsi Kadha Take half liter (500 ml) of water.

- Add few leafs of tulsi around eight to ten leafs.
- Add some Elachi(Cardamom) Powder around half spoon.
- Boil this mixture till it becomes around 250 ml.
- Give this mixture to patient in lukewarm condition.
- It will give relief.

For Asthama

Take tulsi leafs with somr rock salt & chew it. Regular usage will remove asthama.

For Diabetes

Regular eating of Tulsi can keep your blood sugar in control.

For Cold and Cough

Chew tulsi leafs with ginger, in 2 to 3 days, you can get relief from cold and cough.

For Headache

Tulsi can give relief from pain, chew 4 to 5 leafs, it will give relief.

For Stress

Take 10 to 12 leafs in morning & take another 10 to 12 leafs in evening. It will reduce stress. It improves blood circulation in the body.

For Knee Pain

Take tulsi leafs, tulsi seeds & tulsi roots, all three in same proportion. Make its powder, take this mixture with jaggery. It will give relief from pain.

For Eyes

Tulsi has two types shyam tulsi (Dark in colour) & Shwait Tusli (Normal in color). For eyes problem pour two drops of shyam tulsi leafs juice in eyes. It can give relief from any issues of eyes.

For Ear issues

Mix camphor in tulsi juice, make it warm, pour two to three drops in ear, it will give relief from any issues.

For Kidney stones

The main reason is increased quantity of uric acid in blood. Tulsi leafs are very helpful in getting relief from kidney stones. Regular usage is recommended till you get relief.

For Burned Skin

Mix tulsi juice & coconut oil, apply it on burned skin, it will give relief and fast recovery.

For Hair fall

Mix tulsi powder with coconut oil & apply on hair roots. It will give relief.

HEALTH BENEFITS OF TEA, COFFEE & MILK

Tea

Tea is brought to India by BRITISH peoples; tea plants grow especially in cold regions. Tea is medicine only for those peoples who have low blood pressure. Peoples who are living in cold regions like Europe, CANADA, USA & few parts on India like J & K, Himachal, Uttrakhand, peoples from these regions ,generally have low blood pressure, so tea is very useful for them. Tea can give immediate rise in blood pressure.

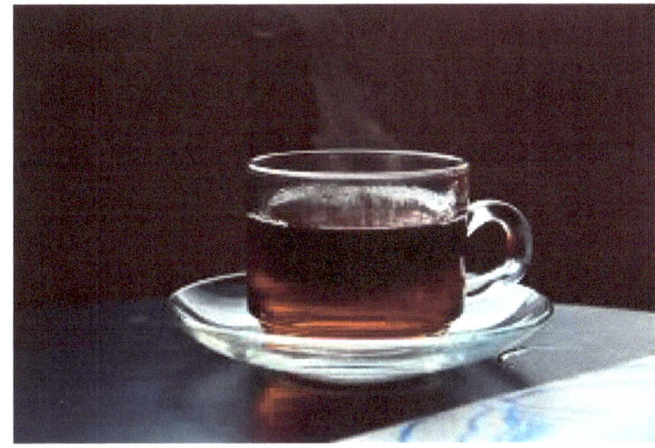

But peoples who stay in hot areas of INDIA like Rajasthan, Maharashtra, Delhi, Tamilnadu etc. & any other hot countries of world. Where temperature is normal or high in summer, most of peoples have normal or high blood pressure. Tea is very harmful for them, if you continue to drink tea for many years in hot areas. It can lead to disease of hypertension. Those who are suffering with high blood pressure, it is recommended that they should stop drinking tea or coffee immediately.

Tea is acidic in nature. Peoples living in cold religions have less acidic blood, so tea helps them to get normal level of acidity. But peoples living in hot areas, if drinks tea, there blood will become more acidic, so it will be harmful for them.

Never take tea with empty stomach, after awakening from sleep. After awakening from sleep, around 2 to 3 glass water should be drink. It will reduce your stomach acidity.

Peoples, who have addiction of tea, if want to leave this habit, they can choose option of Arujn tea (Terminalia Arjuna), it is alkaline in nature. It will help to recover bad effects of tea. In INDIA lot of other herbal tea products are available which are alkaline in nature. Ajwain & Cumin (Hindi word- Jeera) are alkaline in nature, you can make its tea, instead of sugar use jaggery (hindi word Gud).It will also help to reduce acidity of blood and make it neutral.

Coffee

It contains caffeine which is psychoactive, which gives you fresh feeling and energetic. If you drink coffee without sugar (BLACK COFFEE), then it helps to throw out toxin and bacteria.

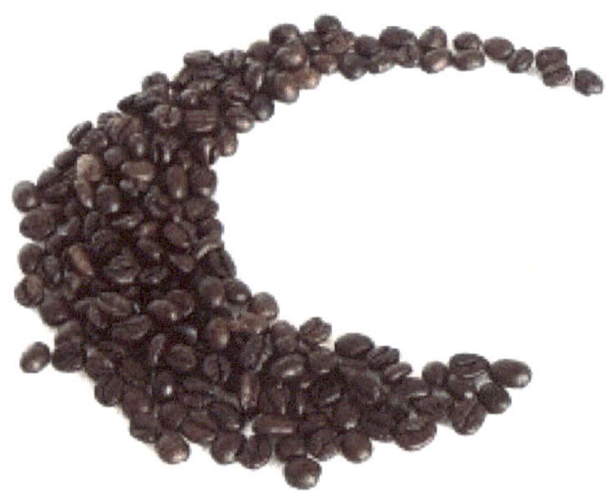

 Black coffee without sugar helps to reduce your weight at a faster rate. Black coffee improves your metabolism by around 50%. It helps to reduce fat & is also helpful for health of your heart. It also helps to reduce body inflation. It have good amount of antioxidants. It also contains vitamins B2, B3, Pro vitamin B5, Magnesium &manganese. It can control type 2 diabetes. It has some anti-cancer properties also.

Black coffee keeps your body and mind healthy. Caffeine increases dopamine, which helps to prevent disease like PARKINSON. A cup of coffee can reduce your body fatigue & also turn your mood to positive and energetic.

Coffee Precautions

1. Do not drink coffee more than 3 to 4 cups a day, it can be harmful to your body.

2. It can reduce your sleep.

3. It can also lead to fear.

4. Pregnant ladies should not drink more than 2 cups of coffee.

Milk

Milk is recommended to drink before sleeping. After sunset it is more beneficial than day time. It recovers your body from fatigue & gives you good sleep. It contains amino acids which improves your Harmon's of sleep. Milk contains calcium, which can lead to stronger bones. Milk also contains proteins, which is useful for our muscles. Milk should not be very hot or very cold. It should be light warm or equivalent to our normal body temperature. If one spoon of ghee is mixed with a glass of milk then, It increases sexual power. As per Ayurveda, milk should be drink after 2 to 3 hours of dinner. Then only you will get full benefits of milk. Do not mix sugar with milk, it reduces calcium, if you need sweet you can mix honey, crystal sugar or raisin (Dry grapes).

Milk & honey if mixed together then it give tremendous benefits. It gives you glowing skin, and healthy body. It improves your immunity.

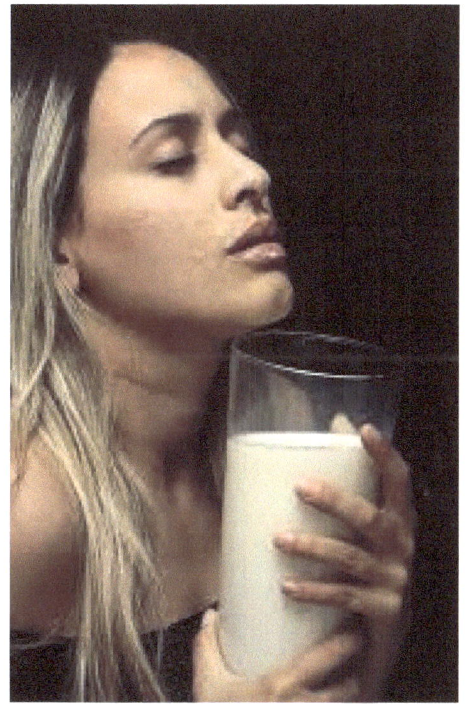

Health Remedy using milk.

Cough

 Milk & turmeric if mixed with each other. Then it can cure cough &cold.

Daily 200 ml of milk and half spoon of turmeric are recommended. You have to boil it, after cooling down you can sip it. It gives relief from cough. It can reduce pain due to injury & also helps to reduce swelling.

Weight & Muscles Improvement

 Take a banana, cut it into small pieces, mix with 200 ml of milk & boil it. After cooling down you can sip it, It also reduces acidity. Helps in weight gain & muscles improvement.

Improvement of Memory

Take 7 pieces of almonds. Make its powder & mix with 200 ml of milk. Boil this mixture; you can add crystal sugar as per need. This kind of milk boost your memory power, gives you health & also useful in dry cough.

Constipation & Anemia

Take 200 ml of milk & 50 gram of Papita (It is fruit in INDIA, it is HINDI word). Mix it in grinder & make its juice. Do not add sugar. You have to drink this juice once in a day. Continuous usage will remove constipation & anemia. It is also helpful in lever disease.

Hemorrhoids & Crush On: Take 200 ml of milk. Taken 10 raisins (Dry Grapes) without seeds, boil this mixture. Take this milk for 15 days before sleeping. It improves immunity & increases blood & helpful in recovery from Hemorrhoids & crush on.

HEALTH BENEFITS OF FLAX SEEDS (अलसी का बीज)

Flax seeds is a rich source of fibers, antioxidants, amino acids, omega 3 fatty acids & minerals. It also contains manganese, magnesium & vitamin B complex. Also contains protein, zinc and calcium.

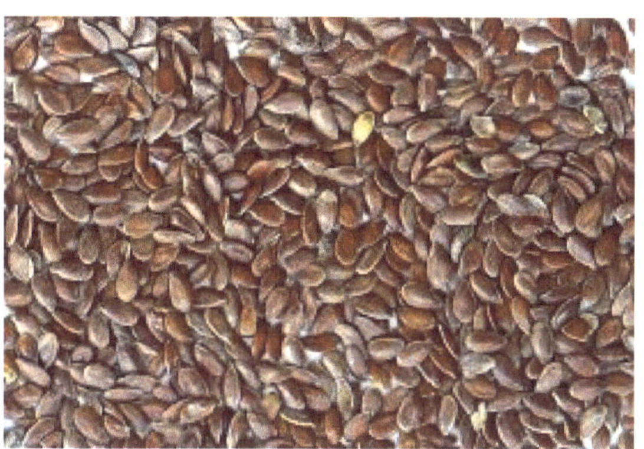

How to eat.

1. It can be directly chewed.
2. It can be roasted.
3. It can be grind as powder, powder gives more benefits than above two.
4. It can be mixed with curds or milk.

Health Benefits

1. It contains soluble & insoluble fibers, which makes our digestive system strong. Helps to remove constipation.
2. Soluble fibers dissolve in water, due to which our stomach remains full, it reduces hunger & It helps in weight loss.
3. Amino acids & omega 3 fatty acids helps to reduce blood pressure. So peoples having high blood pressure should include 2 spoons flax seeds powders in their daily diet.
4. Omega 3 fatty acids give strength to muscles.
5. It also burns extra fat.
6. It is also helpful in heart disease. It prevents hardness of arteries. It also reduces blood clotting.
7. It helps in treatment of irregular heartbeat. It keeps our heat healthy.
8. It increase HDL(Good cholesterol), it reduces LDL (bad cholesterol).

9. It increases insulin sensitivity level in our blood. If 2 spoons of powder is included in our daily food, it improves blood sugar level. It prevents diabetes

10. Antioxidants protects us from breast cancer, colon cancer & prostate cancer. Its antigenic properties prevents growth of tumors.

11. It works as anti-inflammatory agent.

12. It is also helpful for recovery of asthma.

13. It increases overall immunity.

14. It reduces stress level & uplift our mood.

15. It is helpful from recovery of depression.

16. It improves calcium absorption, so gives strengths to our bones & joints. So there is no possibility of joint pain in old age.

17. It improves both male & female fertility.

18. In ladies at the time of menopause, it helps to recover from hot flashes.

19. It also gives health to our skin and hairs. It reduces wrinkles and fine lines. It moisturize our skin. Reduces hair fall. It strength hair roots & removes dandruff.

20. If you mix powders with curds, it can be used as scribe for our face, which can reduce black heads.

Side effects

• Delays blood clotting time. If you have moist stitches or wound on body, do not use flax seeds,

• If we consume more flax seeds, or we do not drink enough water after taking flax seeds, it can create blockage in esophagus.

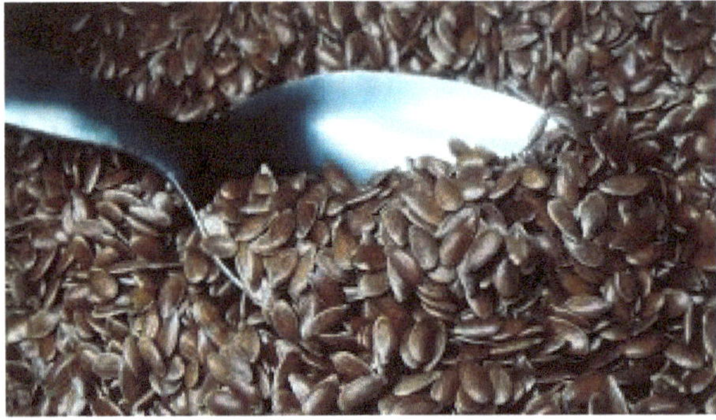

• If we consume more flax seeds, then it can result in loose stool.

• Those peoples which have Ulcerative colitis, diabetic colitis, crohn's disease irritable bowel syndrome, they should not eat flax seeds.

• Lot of use of flax seeds can cause breast & prostate cancer.
• Excessive use can cause allergy includes stomach pain & omitting.
• For ladies excessive use can create problem in conceiving.
• Eating flax seeds is not safe in pregnancy.
• It can increase liquidly of blood, so peoples who are using medicines should not use it.
• Peoples who are using medicines for diabetes and BP, before taking flax seeds, they have to stop medicines or they should consult their physician.
• Ladies who are doing breast feeding for their child , should not use flax seeds.

PANCH KARMA

Panch means five and Karma means actions or therapy to cure various diseases. It is a very advance therapy in Ayurveda. It do not have any side effects like allopathic.

Its main purpose is to remove all type of toxins from body and clean the body. After removing the toxins from the body more than 50% of diseases are cured without any medicines. For remains there is also less needs of medicines.

Before start of panch karma there are two Purva (Prior) Karmas. These are Snehan and Swedan.

Snehan

Snehana means Oleation or to make smooth In this therapy a special oil massage in done on hole body, so that skin can easily throw out toxins from body. In this process toxic substances are liquefied in the body.

Sweadan

In this warm steam is given to body, a special container is used, only head come out of this container, and remaining body is exposed to warm steam. Due to this process body throws out toxic substance through sweat.

Shirodhara

Shirodhara is a form of Ayurveda therapy that involves gently pouring liquids over the forehead and can be one of the steps involved in Panchakarma. The name comes from the Sanskrit words shiro (head) and dhara (flow). The liquids used in shirodhara depend on what is being treated, but can include oil, milk, buttermilk, coconut water, or even plain water.

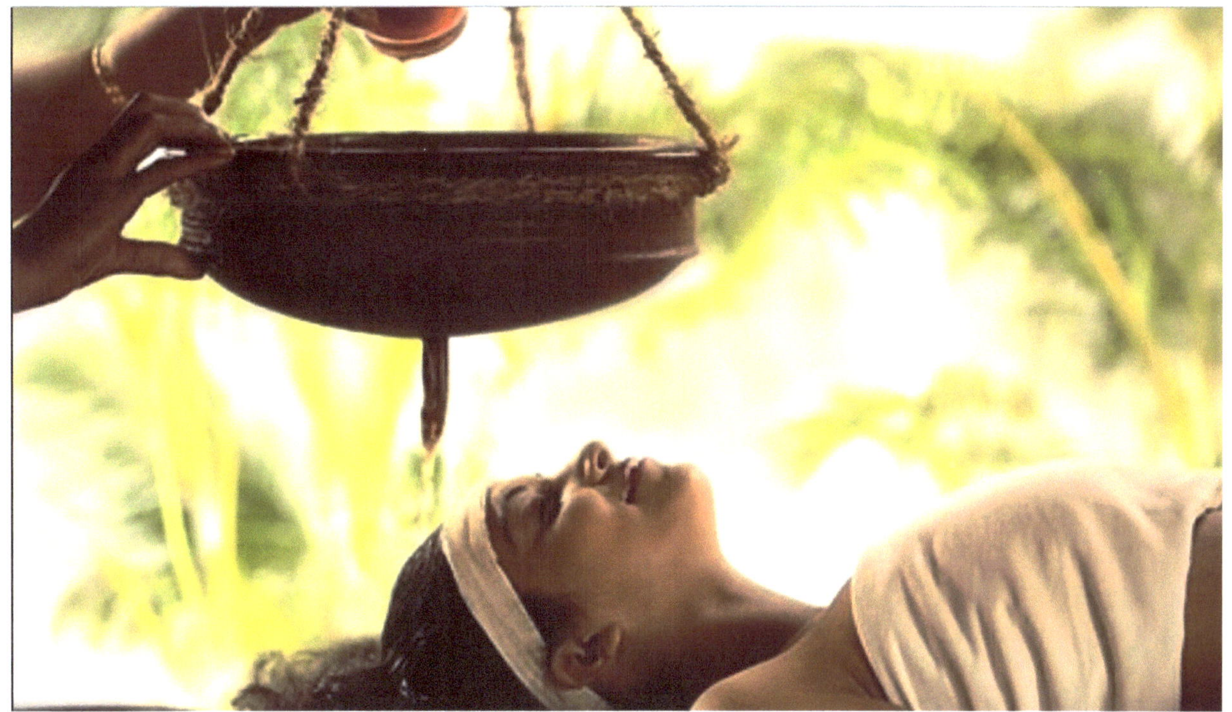

Shirodhara has been used to treat a variety of conditions including eye diseases, mental disease, sinusitis, allergic rhinitis, greying of hair, neurological disorders, memory loss, insomnia, hearing impairment, tinnitus, vertigo, Meniere's disease and certain types of skin diseases like psoriasis. It is also used non-medicinally at spas for its relaxing properties. Studies report that Ayurvedic Shirodhara is a safe option to improve sleep quality among people who have sleep problems. Shirodhara is also effective in treating mental conditions such as anxiety, and mental stress. The calming effect produced by Shirodhara is similar to that obtained with meditation.

Panchkarma & Shirodhar together becomes shatkarma (six therapy).

After this Panch Karma Starts. Which are as below.

1. Waman
2. Basti
3. Nasaya
4. Rakta Mokshan (Blood Purification)
5. Virechan

Waman

It is used for frequent cough, cold and asthama. In this therapy mixture of honey and mulethi is given to patient ,after that patient rub his tongue & try to omit , due to which omitting occurs & it throws out toxins from the body.

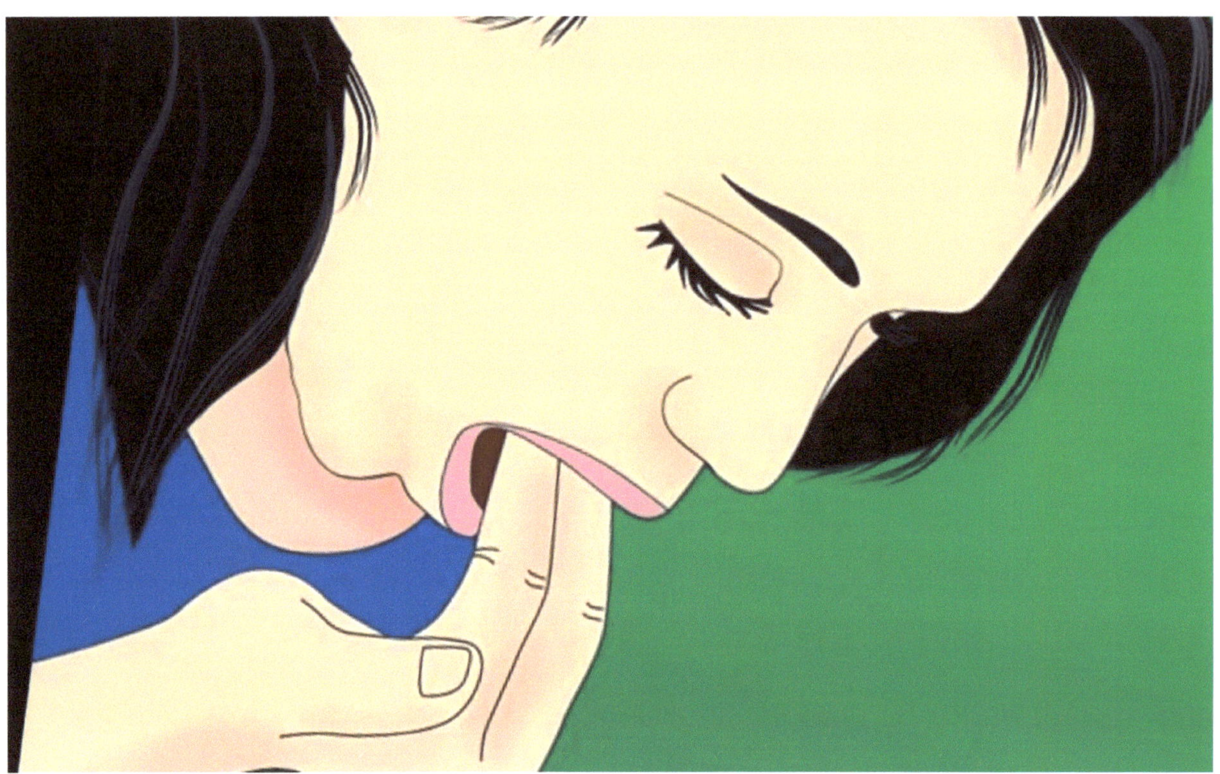

This process is repeated for 4 to 8 times. And after this patient get immediate relief from kapha.

Basti

It is used for diseases like constipation, diabetes ,paralyses ,arthritis, joint pen etc. In this therapy all toxins occurred due to vata, pitta and kapha are thrown out through anus. For it some medicine oil are injected though anus, for which special machines are used.

Nasaya

In this therapy nose passage are cleaned with help of medicines. Some drops of medicine are poured in nose & through nose only toxins are thrown out. It is used for disease related to brain, headache, migraine, cynocytic etc.

Rakta Mokshan

It is used for skin disease like leprosy. In this process small wounds are made on skin at various places, so that it can throw out blood. At some places small worms are used, which can suck blood of patient.

Virechan

The Virachana therapy is medicated purification therapy, cleansing the body from excess pitta accumulation, purifying blood and clearing toxins. The therapy primarily concentrates on the toxins accumulated in the liver and gall bladder, thus cleansing the gastro-intestinal tract completely.

In Virechana detoxification therapy, vitiated doshas and toxins are eliminated through the rectum. The therapy involves intake of Ayurvedic and herbal medicines that destroy the doshas and toxin from the body and bring them to the abdomen. Since Pitta is situated at the level of intestines, it is best to expel it from the anal route. The Ayurvedic medicines used for the therapy may vary from person to person depending on the patient's digestion strength. During the Virechana Ayurvedic treatment, the patient will be subjected to oral intake of Ayurvedic medicines followed by fermentation. The patient will also be subjected to a personalized light and warm diet.

Virechana Therapy is recommended and is highly beneficial for the following:

- Detoxification in case of accumulation of Pitta dosha,
- Eliminates toxin accumulation in the GI tract,
- Effective treatment for piles, constipation, acidity, ulcers, liver, spleen diseases, jaundice, inflammations,
- Cleanses body from poisoning,
- Cures mild and chronic skin disorders,
- Reduces gynaecological disorders

- Relives headaches, anemia, pain in the large intestine, non-healing wounds- Helps manage diabetes, asthma and heart diseases.